STRUCTURE OF LIFESTYLE

A Rising Sun to a New Life.
Live Medication Free

by
Allen Richman

Bloomington, IN  Milton Keynes, UK

authorHOUSE™

AuthorHouse™
1663 Liberty Drive, Suite 200
Bloomington, IN 47403
www.authorhouse.com
Phone: 1-800-839-8640

AuthorHouse™ UK Ltd.
500 Avebury Boulevard
Central Milton Keynes, MK9 2BE
www.authorhouse.co.uk
Phone: 08001974150

First published by AuthorHouse 2/6/2006

ISBN: 1-4259-1269-9 (sc)

Library of Congress Control Number: 2006900059

Printed in the United States of America
Bloomington, Indiana

This book is printed on acid-free paper.

TO MY EVER-INSPIRING, LOVELY WIFE
MARICAR

TABLE OF CONTENTS

THE KEY AND HOW TO OPEN THE DOOR

In all human beings, we have one thing in common!

Physiologically we are basically all the same.

So if this statement is true, then in order to teach people how to obtain good health, can become a non-confining area of life.

To further explain, we must realize that the most important function of the body, sitting at the very throne of all functions of the body, is the immune system.

Now stop and think, if we have a strong immune system, then what are the conditions of all the body's major organs that control all systems of the body and its vital functions?

When all of the body's vital functions are working in excellent condition, we feel, act, think, and perform at a level of radiant health. At this level, stress rolls off us like water on a duck's back. We don't even recognize stress as a problem at all, and many other conditions of everyday life become a joy.

Remember this phrase:

Without change, nothing is possible and with change, anything is possible.

THE CHOICE IS YOURS.
ONLY YOU CAN BE RESPONSIBLE FOR
YOUR OWN HEALTH.
NO ONE ELSE!!!

CHAPTER I

REGENERATION OR DEGENERATION

There was a time when conversation between friends was about family, sports, cars, vacations, hopes and dreams, politics, your occupation, or religion. Today, the main topic of conversation seems to be about our latest health problem: how sick we are, how tired we are, how crummy we feel, our aches and pains, our lack of energy...etc, etc, etc.

Something has gone wrong! The facts indicate a natural health crisis is upon us. What are our choices? Are there solutions? One thing is certain: we cannot drug ourselves into health. If this was so, we would be a healthy nation by now. However, there is an answer, but it requires you to personally take charge of your health. No one else can do it for you.

THE CHOICE IS YOURS
What is Health?

We all want good health, but what is it? Health is not merely an absence of illness. It is evidenced by a steady state of euphoria and positive well-being. This is rarely experienced by humans today.

The people we meet can be divided into four groups:
1. People who are definitely sick.
2. People who are almost sick.
3. People who think they are healthy.
4. People who are experiencing a high level of health.

Most of us will find ourselves in one of the first three groups. A very small percentage of our population will be in the fourth category. Being filled with the joy of living, an overflowing energy, and an overall feeling of well-being is a very rare experience for most people today.

True health involves painless, sound bodily movements; efficiently working vital organs; and mental faculties operating at full throttle. Much of our well-being stems from our heredity, but this is only our starting point for building and maintaining optimum health.

Health is easily seen in others. They radiate superior health. Their eyes are clear and seem to sparkle with life. There is clearness and a living color to their skin. They have a bounce in their step and their joyful feeling for life is infectious. You are excited to be around them. Their health is like a bubbling fountain within. A zeal for life, enthusiasm, joy, bountiful energy, and a "natural high" for life characterizes health. But, we rarely see this kind of exuberant physiological masterpiece walking around in the U.S.A. today.

This vitality can be achieved for most of us during our three score and ten (if the damage we have done to ourselves is not beyond the point of no return). All of this can be ours, but we must seek it. Good health cannot be produced by our unhealthy living practices.

To fail or refuse to seek health will rob us of everything good. Without health, the opportunity or the potential each of us was born with will never have a chance to develop to its full potential. We could even become a burden to those we love the most.

> *WHEN HEALTH IS ABSENT,*
> *WISDOM CANNOT REVEAL ITSELF,*
> *ART CANNOT BECOME MANIFEST,*
> *STRENGTH CANNOT BE EXERTED,*
> *WEALTH BECOMES USELESS,*
> *AND REASON IS POWERLESS.*

HEROPHILUS, 300 B.C.

THE CONDITIONS FOR HEALTH

Our requirements for good health are almost identical to those of a plant. We need fresh air, pure drinking water, sunshine, nourishing food, and warmth. Without these, both plants and humans will perish. These are the bare essentials of life. If we restrict ourselves to only one of these, we will die. Our health is determined by our use or abuse of these five basic requirements of life.

The additional five balancing factors for health are exercise, proper sanitation, rest and sleep, emotional fulfillment, and a purpose for living. These ten prerequisites for life are the conditions for our good health. The lack of any of these can be the cause of our poor health.

All of the factors are so interdependent that none can stand alone or be complete without the others.

THE CAUSES OF HEALTH

Just as there are causes of disease, there are also causes of health.

Each day our bodies heal themselves with the raw materials ingested. This healing process takes place on a microscopic level, and the success or failure of healing also depends on the quality of these raw materials (food).

We are never as intelligent as the body. It regulates the chemistry of its fluids and tissues and knows exactly what to do and when to do it. We must rely on this automatic mechanism to correct all the injustices we impose on ourselves.

There are laws of health that are just as reliable and immutable as the law of gravity, the laws of thermodynamics, and all the other physical laws of the universe.

A fundamental healing principle is:

All cells act to preserve themselves at all times.

This instinct is sustained by a "vital force" or life. The success of this force is directly proportionate to the amount or strength of it. While individual cells attempt to preserve themselves, they are working together to preserve the whole.

When we understand the grandeur of the body's defense mechanisms, used to maintain cellular purity, we may come to the astounding revelation that we really have to work hard to inflict ourselves with sickness.

About now you are probably wondering, "How can I regain my health when sick and stay healthy when I'm well?" The answer is not something mysterious, complicated, or hard to understand. The answer is two-fold.

1. Remove all causes of disease
2. Supply the conditions for health

Like weeds in a garden, the causes of disease must be removed. If we first do not remove these causes, our health improvement is impossible. Would you try to heal a burn by continually burning yourself? If you want the burn to heal, you must remove the flame.

THE CAUSES OF DISEASE

1. Excesses
2. Deficiencies
3. Poor Emotional Habits
4. Poison Habits

1. EXCESSES

Our excesses are acts that exceed the normal things in our life. Some of the more common excesses are overeating, overdrinking (any liquid), taking baths too often, overworking, too much sun, too much exercise, too much sleep, and being too emotional.

All of these are normal factors in life. They just need to be supplied in proper quantity and quality in order to restore and preserve health.

Any excesses have an enervating effect on the body and, as such, are the very beginning cause of disease.

2. DEFICIENCIES

The soil our food is grown in is not in the same condition it was one hundred years ago. It has become depleted of the minerals needed for healthy plants, which provide us the nutrition for body maintenance and healing.

This depletion has been caused by erosion, not replacing the organic matter to the soil, failure to rotate crops, and never allowing the land to rest. Added to these natural depletions are the unnatural ones. These include artificial fertilizers, herbicides to control weeds, fungicides to control fungi, and pesticides to control insects. All of these end up in our food.

Our preparation of this food decreases even further whatever available nutrients are left in the food. We cook it and destroy the living enzymes. We nuke it with micro-waves, which alter the molecular structure. We blast it with radiation to give it a longer shelf life. We denature our food and then try to make it wholesome again by adding back what we think it needs in the form of synthetic vitamins (from coal tar). We process and package our food so that it can sit on a shelf for months and not spoil.

After all this, we—in our great wisdom—play chemist with our bodies, try to guess what we need, and rely on vitamins and minerals in pill form (all synthetic and without life) to replace what has been taken or destroyed in our food.

To regain and maintain our health we must eat whole natural foods, prepared in their natural state before they have been changed in any way. Your main source of food should consist of fruits, vegetables, nuts, seeds, and food-grade herbs. All should be organically grown, if possible. This is the best way for us to receive the nourishment needed for maintenance and healing.

Our other deficiencies are too little sleep, insufficient exercise, lack of sunshine, no friends or interpersonal relationships, or a lack of emotional fulfillment.

A deficiency in any one of these normal needs of life can also be enervating and a remote or basic cause of disease.

3. POOR EMOTIONAL HABITS

Your emotional habits can cause disease just as much as eating unhealthy foods. Detrimental emotional habits are formed from birth. Poor environment, unhealthy family relations, or even being allowed to feel sorry for yourself and wallow in self-pity will take its toll on your health.

It doesn't really matter how or why we may have an emotional habit. What counts is recognizing the problem and then proceeding to do something about it. These emotional handicaps can be smashed just as we can overcome poor physical habits. Sometimes, in order to make a dramatic, dynamic lasting breakthrough, professional counseling or confiding in a very close friend may be needed.

We are all human. We all make mistakes. **Probably the most important ingredient for emotional health is the ability to forgive.**

Our first step toward changing poor emotional habits is realizing they exist. Hatred, anger, wrath, strife, envy, jealousy, lust, greed, worry, anxiety, resentment, selfishness, self-centeredness, self-pity, and being argumentative, introverted, overly critical, unforgiving, and unfriendly all have negative physiological consequences on our bodies.

One very dominant trend in our society is to suffer from extremely low self-esteem. Each of us carries far too much emotional baggage around in his or her head. Every individual is unique and has something special to offer. You will never find it until you look. For starters, try to be encouraging to others.

These negative personality traits or emotions have varied effects on our health, but the common denominator is their tendency to paralyze normal body functions (cellular metabolism).

When we continue any of these poor emotions, metabolic wastes are not properly eliminated and negative pathological changes take place.

Our emotions can be so enervating that one emotional upset may fatigue us to the point that it may take weeks to recover from this tremendous expenditure of nerve energy.

PROGRESS IS IMPOSSIBLE WITHOUT CHANGE; AND THOSE WHO CANNOT CHANGE THEIR MINDS CANNOT CHANGE ANYTHING.

GEORGE BERNARD SHAW

FRIENDS MAY HELP
KEEP DISEASE AWAY.

People who value power over friendship may have a harder time fighting off disease and get sick more often, new research suggests.

But having supportive friendships can boost immune function and help fight disease —even under stress.

Studies by Princeton University psychologist John B. Jemmott III add to growing evidence that personality can affect ability to fight illness. He looked at immune function at times of high and low stress for 257 men and women.

Some valued relationships and socializing, others were strongly power-driven—assertive, competitive, focused on collecting status symbols or promotions. Among key findings:

During high-stress periods, those with lots of friendships had significantly higher levels of IGA—part of the immune system that helps fight infection, particularly upper respiratory infections.

Under stress, they also had significantly higher activity among cells that recognize and kill tumors and viruses.

Power-driven people took longer to recover normal IGA levels of stress.

Those with the toughest shield: unstressed people with active social lives.

One explanation: power-driven personalities may produce more adrenaline, which suppresses immune function.

4. POISON HABITS

If a substance is not required and is never used physiologically, then it is in reality a poison. Any amount is a poison, no matter how small.

An obvious example is smoking. There is no bodily requirement for smoke and the more than 200 chemicals that are inhaled in the smoke. The body simply does not use any part of the smoke for building tissue or maintaining body fluids.

Any food that has a substance in it or on it that is not a food becomes a poison. These include any foods with preservatives, artificial colorings, artificial sweeteners, etc. Especially damaging are soft drinks, and foods with processed white sugar or salt.

Health cannot be achieved while we are poisoning ourselves. Some of these habits may be hard to break because they are addictive. But these are weeds that must be removed from your garden. These habits may be removed abruptly or slowly, but they must be removed if you really plan to reach your goal of superior health.

Think on this! No responsible chemist would mix all of the chemicals we take into our bodies every day. No study has ever been done on the chemical interactions that take place between all of these chemicals. We are creating a Pandora's chemist pot within us.

HEALTH DESTROYERS

- Aluminum

- Antibiotics in your Meat

- Antibiotics in your Milk

- Artificial Coloring

- Artificial Flavors

- BHA

- BHT

- Bleached Flour

- Chlorinated Water

- Cigarettes

- Drugs

- Fluoridated Water

- Heavy Metals

- Herbicides and Fungicides

- High Fat Diet

- Irradiated Food

- MSG

- Pesticides

- Salt

- Soda

- Sodium Nitrite

- Synthetic Vitamins

- Too Much Alcohol

- White Sugar

HOW AND WHY SYMPTOMS APPEAR

When we become sick, we should not think in terms of the name of the disease but instead realize the entire body is infected or affected—not just the location of the problem. All diseases are only local manifestations of an overall toxic system. Simply put, the body chemistry is out of balance.

Our illnesses start with enervation (to deprive of nerve, force, or strength) that leads to toxicosis or toxemia (an over-accumulation of toxins within the body, or "blood poisoning").

Our body operates on nerve energy. If this energy is sufficiently replaced through rest and sleep and we are fulfilling the laws or causes of health, we will remain healthy.

However, if our outgoing energy exceeds the replacement of energy, we will experience enervation. Our deficient diet and other negative living habits will catch up with us. Our body may not be able to keep up with the expulsion of the byproducts of metabolism. When these toxins, plus those we take in with our food and water, rise above our personal tolerance level, the body—out of self-preservation—initiates an elimination process. We get sick.

The symptoms can vary from person to person. It depends on which part of our body is a weak point and where our quickest exit point of toxic material may be.

Even though the symptoms of a particular disease can be unpleasant, it is evidence the body is making an attempt at cleaning house. Healing and purification are beginning to take place. To suppress this bodily response, or cleansing, would be a mistake. Continued suppression prevents the body from cleansing itself, and the toxins are retained.

As we continue a devitalizing lifestyle, new toxins are added to the old toxins. The body's filtration systems become even more burdened. Continued suppression inhibits any attempt at cleansing, and the toxins are stored in various parts of the body. Eventually the level of toxicity becomes so intense that the body moves into the next stage of disease.

Should we continue to mask the symptoms with substitution (ignoring the cause and treating only the effects); we are increasing the possibility of reaching the seventh stage of disease ... CANCER.

THERE ARE SOME REMEDIES
WORSE THAN THE DISEASE.

PUBLIUS SYRUS 50 B.C.

THE SEVEN STAGES OF DISEASE

1. ENERVATION

This is a state of nervous exhaustion. The body does not generate enough nerve energy to perform cellular metabolism. Nerve energy is a form of electricity measurable in millivolts. When there is too little of it, body functions become impaired, including getting rid of wastes.

2. TOXEMIA

The accumulation of debris from the normal cellular breakdown of dead cells and the addition of external toxins has reached a level too great for the body to handle. In an attempt at self-preservation, the body cleans house by ridding itself of the toxins. During this process we are sick with cold or flu symptoms.

3. IRRITATION

The nerve network senses toxic materials. We feel irritation in the areas affected by toxic wastes. This is an alarm that something is wrong.

4. INFLAMMATION

You are keenly aware that there is a problem. It involves pain. The body begins to redirect its vital energies. The intestinal tract is shut down. We give these diseases names that end in "it is," such as tonsillitis, appendicitis, colitis, etc. Inflammation is the body's response to a life-threatening situation. This is the body's most intensive effort to cleanse and restore itself.

5. ULCERATION

This is a degenerative stage. Due to a toxic system grossly out of balance, staggering amounts of tissue structures are being destroyed. The body cannot cope with the large amounts of toxic material. A void is created where tissues die.

6. INDURATION

The voids are filled with toxic material encapsulated by a sac of hardened tissue. Toxic material sealed off in this manner is called a tumor. This is the last stage of the body's attempt at intelligent control. If we continue the same pathogenic practices that caused the toxemia, this tumorous tissue system goes wild and becomes parasitic, living off nutrients from the lymph system.

7. CANCER

These cells are not capable of organized intelligent direction. They have become disorganized and their genetic coding is altered. Cancer cells flourish and spread as long as nutrients are available, the immune system is out of balance, and we refuse to remove all causes of disease and supply the conditions for health.

Remember: there is a point of no return.

REGENERATION:
THE PROCESS OF PURIFICATION

ALL CURE STARTS FROM WITHIN, THEN MOVING OUTWARD, FROM THE HEAD DOWN AND IN REVERSE ORDER, AS THE SYMPTOMS HAVE APPEARED.

HERING'S LAW OF CURE

FOOD FOR THOUGHT

Most new ideas are usually rejected with varying degrees of skepticism by those who are satisfied with their present circumstances. They are comfortable with their health belief system and see no need for any change on their part. Should they close their minds and throw away the key simply because a concept or idea is new to them? In many cases, what appears new is historically very old. The knowledge is either lost, suppressed, or just now becoming available. Just because the so-called "educated" may laugh, ridicule, and then reject a truth does not make that truth a lie.

IF ANY MAN CAN CONVINCE ME AND BRING HOME TO ME THAT I DO NOT THINK OR ACT ARIGHT, GLADLY WILL I CHANGE; FOR I SEARCH AFTER TRUTH, BY WHICH MAN NEVER YET WAS HARMED. BUT HE IS HARMED WHO ABIDES ON STILL IN HIS DECEPTION AND IGNORANCE.

MARCUS AURELIUS ANTONTUS

At the beginning of the twenty-first century, we still don't have a national interest or incentive to prevent disease. It is a sad truth that 90 percent of our population is merely interested in getting by and oblivious to the fact that they are committing a slow suicide every waking moment. They do not become interested in health until they lose it, or until their jobs are hindered. It is at this point that they begin looking for something to cure or remedy their condition. The solution that most are looking for is a quick-fix ("give me a shot, Doc!"). Then they continue to abuse their bodies with the same injustices that caused their disease in the first place. When such patients' doctors have given up, they at last awaken to the seriousness of their problem and are finally frightened enough to start doing something about it. Unfortunately, it may be too late.

Wouldn't it be better to seek health as a part of your lifestyle? **We basically have two choices. We can pay now for higher quality food or we can pay a whole lot more later (in money and misery) just trying to stay alive.**

FOOD FOR BODY

Before vitality, superior health, overcoming sickness, higher energy levels, or longevity can be achieved, we must begin eating nutrient-dense foods. These are real foods that are never the result of a processing activity. These foods are in the raw state and are electromagnetically charged with a "life force" that is separate and distinct from the caloric energy that is released from food by digestion, enzymatic action, and assimilation. We must be eating whole, natural, and enzyme active foods that have not been refined, processed, overcooked, or preserved with chemicals. These actions, plus microwaving and the new problem of food irradiation with Cobalt-60 and Cestrum 137, render our foods lifeless and devoid of any enzyme activity.

ALL LIFE PROCESSES DEPEND ON ENZYME FUNCTION. WHEN ENZYMES ARE DEPLETED, SO IS OUR VITAL FORCE AND HEALTH.

ENZYMES ARE INVOLVED IN MOVING OUR HANDS AND LEGS, AND EVEN IN THE PROCESS OF THINKING. IF ENZYMES WERE LOST, ALL THE FUNCTIONS OF OUR BODY WOULD FAIL.

Take a sunflower seed and boil it in water. Plant it in fertile soil next to a raw sunflower seed. The concept of bio-energetic nutrition (the electromagnetic or vibrational qualities of living food) now becomes real, as only the raw and unheated seed will sprout. Life begets life.

If we continue to eat food in its unnatural state, we will deplete our bodies' supply of enzymes, which will result in the degeneration of our genetically weaker glands and organs.

**EAT LIVE FOOD TO LIVE;
EAT DEAD FOOD TO DIE.**

WHAT IS THE SOURCE OF YOUR NUTRIENT-DENSE BIO-ENERGETIC FOODS?

In order for Regeneration to take place, the chemical building blocks of life must be made available.

The body requires superior nutrition that is organically grown and free from pesticides, preservatives, or other man-made additives. This type of food is available from a few health food stores. Distance, seasonal selection, spoilage, and the retail cost are all inhibiting and restricting factors.

THE IMPORTANCE OF WATER

The role water plays within our bodies covers five functions: a solvent, transporter, lubricant, coolant, and as a dispersant.

In order for Regeneration to take place without unnecessary hindrances, only pure water should be consumed. Drinking chlorinated, fluoridated, or well water only adds more toxins and impurities for your body to deal with.

It is not the purpose of this book to prove or disprove the merits of drinking only pure, distilled water. There are many books written on this subject. One of these are *The Truth About Water* by Paul Bragg.

THE GREATEST FUNCTION OF DISTILLED WATER

Distilled water acts as a solvent in the body. It dissolves food substances so they can be assimilated and taken into every cell of the body; it dissolves the wastes of cell life so that those poisons and toxins can be carried away from the cells. It dissolves the inorganic mineral substances lodged in tissues of the body so that such substances can be eliminated in the process of purifying the body.

Distilled water is the greatest solvent on earth—the only one that can be taken into the body without damage to the tissues.

By its continued consumption, it is possible to dissolve minerals, acid crystals, and all other waste products of the body without injuring the tissues.

SICKNESS AND DISEASE DO NOT JUST HAPPEN...THEY ACCUMULATE!
THE HEALING CRISIS

A healing crisis is the result of an intense effort of every organ in the body to eliminate waste products and set the stage for Regeneration. Through this reconstructive process toward a healthy body, old inferior tissues are replaced with new superior tissues.

In a healing crisis, there is usually a fever and a catarrhal elimination. These wastes are now in a dissolved free-flowing state, ready to be efficiently removed from the body.

This experience will seem like having disease because of re-experiencing disease symptoms. But there is a very important distinction: elimination. All the eliminative organs are functioning, right up to the time of the crisis. These processes will become more acute because of the abundance of stored energy.

The healing crisis can come without warning. Usually you will feel at your very best shortly before the crisis. The vital forces and energies must become strong enough to initiate these explosive powers of cleansing. Tissue that has been built from poor nutrition and bad living habits will someday have to wrestle with new healthy tissue created from living food.

There are three stages a person must pass through in order to become well:

1. ELIMINATIVE
2. TRANSITIONAL
3. BUILDING

The crisis usually occurs during the transitional period, which is the time when new tissue has become strong enough to function as a more perfect body.

WHEN TO EXPECT A HEALING CRISIS

When the use of stimulants such as coffee, tea, soda pop, and chocolate are suddenly stopped, a headache may occur. This is due to the circulation and discarding of stored toxins called caffeine and theobromine. A letdown will follow due to a heartbeat that is slower because it is no longer being stimulated by the caffeine and theobromine from chocolate. After a few days, these symptoms will go away, and you will feel more energy due to the recuperation that follows.

Eliminating or dramatically cutting back on stimulating animal foods such as meat, fowl, fish, cheeses, milk, eggs, etc., will also result in a slower heartbeat. This may be detected as a state of relaxation or decrease in energy. This initial letdown usually lasts about ten days and is followed by an increase of strength and energy, a feeling of greater well-being, and reduced stress.

When the quality of food and water coming into the body is greater than the tissues the body is made of, the body begins a process of discarding the lower-grade tissues and producing superior-grade cells or tissues.

It may take about three months until the body has the stored energy to start the process. A healing crisis usually lasts about three days, starting with slight pains and discomfort which may become more severe until complete elimination of the toxins has been reached. If the energy level is low, the crisis may last for a week or more.

The more vitality one has, the more powerful the effect of the crisis will be.

THE BODY RESPONSE TO A HEALING CRISIS

During the healing crisis, there is an absence of appetite. The body needs more water to help carry off the toxins that have finally reached the elimination stage. It is also a time for rest. You must rest it out. This includes mental as well as physical rest.

There is not only a physical healing crisis, but a mental crisis as well. We must also have our mental fixations and complexes cleared out of the mind. This is just as important as a cleansing of the bowel or any other organ. If there is a mental state that is causing irritation or colitis in the bowel, the best colonic cannot cure it. Everything must be considered in the build-up to a healing crisis.

When eating, eat only foods that assist in the elimination process—and only small amounts. These foods should be of the type that is easily digested. To eat hard-to-digest food would take away energy that is needed for cleansing and elimination.

STEPS TO REGENERATION

1. THE BODY MUST HAVE A HEALTHY BLOOD STREAM

What flows in the arteries determines whether the body is getting what it needs. Vital living foods must be taken into the body and be properly digested and assimilated.

2. BLOOD MUST CIRCULATE RAPIDLY

Cell structures must be supplied the vital nutrients for regeneration as rapidly as possible.

3. REST

Rest allows the body to recuperate and regenerate. Tiredness is a barometer of our health, and fatigue is the first symptom of all disease. If we don't recognize this alarm, we are abusing ourselves with the greatest hindrance to recovery.

Regeneration will take place when superior tissue is exchanged for the old tissue by the blood stream.

ANY DIET, IN ORDER TO BE EFFECTIVE FOR HEALING AND BODY CLEANSING, MUST CONSIST OF FOODS THAT CONTAIN NOT MERELY THE RECOGNIZED "FOOD VALUES," BUT THE INHERENT QUALITIES NECESSARY FOR CLEANSING, HEALING, AND FOR THE ELIMINATION OF POISONOUS WASTES.

THE RETRACING PROCESS

All healing in the body starts from within and works outward, from the head down, and in the reverse order that the diseases and injuries in your life have appeared.

The body, in its great wisdom and innate intelligence, automatically heals the most serious problem first. Fortunately, we don't have to consciously make that decision.

The intelligence within your body knows more about tissue structure and repair, (Regeneration), than any scientist or doctor will ever know.

This retracing process is really a very just process when we consider that our living habits and the foods we eat ultimately determine what we are (You are what you eat; you are what you think).

Usually people do not remember what diseases or injuries they may have had in the past, but during the healing crisis, they are reminded of what they have forgotten.

By going back through all of the health problems that we have caused and inflicted upon ourselves, we are really burning into our brain the realization of cause and effect. By re-experiencing our past health problems, we are learning the importance of taking care of ourselves. We are also learning that there is a penalty for the "sins of the flesh." Sometimes, but not always, the discomfort during the healing crisis or retracing may be more notable than while we were building the chronic disease. But this is for only a short time. Always look to the goal of total health and freedom from disease. Even more importantly, you will now be able to encourage others.

Once we retrace back to health, we will become so completely converted to honoring the laws of health that we will never want to go back to the ways that cause disease.

HOW TO TELL THE DIFFERENCE BETWEEN A HEALING CRISIS AND A DISEASE CRISIS

HEALING CRISIS

- A blessing to the body.

- Just before the crisis you feel great with energy to spare.

- It is brought on by an accumulation of health.

- All organs are acutely eliminating waste products and setting the stage for Regeneration.

- Many parts of the body show marked change and improvement.

- Absence of appetite.

The crisis may be as simple as a rash, pimple, or boils.

Elimination is regular right up to the time of the crisis. Usually a fever or catarrhal elimination takes place. Stored wastes are now in a dissolved, free-flowing state, and a cleansing purifying action is under way.

It will take place about three months after you have begun making serious changes in your lifestyle.

It will last 3 to 7 days, depending on your personal energy level.

DISEASE CRISIS

- A curse on the body.

- You feel progressively worse before you become sick.

- It is brought on by toxemia.

- Every organ works against it, rather that with it, as in the healing crisis.

- Only part of the body shows any marked change or improvement.

- Just before it, there is often a tremendous increase in appetite for all the wrong foods—especially sugar products.

- There are no simple disease crises.

- Elimination is shut down or is very unsatisfactory.

It may take years before your body reacts to your abuse. The longer it takes, the more serious the problem.

The disease crisis can last for weeks and months, depending on how abused your body is, especially if you continue doing what caused the problem in the first place.

CHRONOLOGY OF A HEALING CRISIS: HOW WE RETRACE

HEALTH

2 years old: Acute Stage of Disease

(Frequent Colds)

10 years old: Sub-Acute Stage of Disease

(Flu & Bronchial Disorders)

28 years old: Chronic Stage of Disease

(Hay Fever, Pneumonia)

38 years old: Sub-Chronic Stage of Disease

(Asthma, Rheumatism)

Any Age: Degenerative Stage of Disease

(Cancer, MS, Arthritis, etc.)

Regeneration is dependent upon cleansing of the bodily tissues and replacing the old tissues with new cells. In the reversal process of chronic disease, sometimes past diseases recur just the same as they were previously developed. We cannot put a new foundation in the body without first cleansing the body, a process that is not always comfortable. Those who have lived better lives in the past, who have eaten better foods, and who have abused their bodies less with overeating will have very mild or almost no bodily responses. Those who have poisoned themselves with "food" created by modern food processing will have more pronounced symptoms, if they have damaged the eliminating organs. When these organs have regenerated to a healthy, more efficient state, they will no longer produce the symptoms of disease.

CHAPTER II

FOODS TO AVOID
DURING THE HEALING PROCESS

Avoid all meats except wild Alaska salmon and eggs for your protein source. Also avoid all dairy products, sweets, honey, natural syrups, sucrose, fructose, white/brown and raw sugars.

Avoid all fruits, including bananas and avocados, canned or bottled fruit juices, and vegetable juices. Avoid soft drinks (carbonated), coffee, and tea (except for certain herbal beverages). Avoid these vegetables: potato, tomato, eggplant, asparagus, spinach, beet, and sweet potato. Sugar content of fruits—bananas, mangos (highest) and grapefruit (lowest). Overripe fruit should be avoided.

Look toward grains and other vegetables for a good source of protein, such as adzuki beans, millet, and brown rice.

I highly recommend leaning toward a vegetarian diet, especially during the healing process. If you must eat meat later on, eat it in moderation (fish and turkey only). Eat no deli foods, or any food with preservatives or any chemicals. Drink only distilled water. Do not eat leftovers in the fridge that are more than eight hours old.

Eliminate all canned foods. Tuna in water is all right. Eliminate all processed and refined foods. Eat short-grain brown rice daily. A great percentage of your diet should be brown rice during the healing process.

Best source of Omega 3 oils are ground flax seed, to powder and mix in unsweetened soy milk. Combine three to four tablespoons of ground flax seed with one Stevia Extract packet. Stevia will naturally lower blood sugar levels and give you more energy. Protein and heavy meals taken later in the daytime or evening will inhibit sound sleep. Before bed, Light carbohydrate meals will improve sleep.

Avoid foods containing yeast. Food will develop yeast in your refrigerator if it is there for too long.

HARMFUL FOODS WITH YEAST

- Mushrooms – Bread – Pastries

- Truffles

- Cheese

- Butter – Milk – Flour (enriched from yeast)

- Cottage Cheese

- Vinegars (Apple, Gin, Pear, Grape, and Distilled)

- Catsup

- Mayonnaise

- Olives

- Pickles

- Sauerkraut

- Condiments

- Horseradish

- Salad Dressings

- Barbeque Sauce

- Tomato Sauce

- Chili Peppers

- Mince Pie

- Liquor and Wine

- Malted Products

- Candies

After healing, if you encounter backsliding (your old ways), it won't take you very long to realize what you must do to recapture and regain control of your health.

Remember: Whatever the illness, it did not happen overnight. You might think otherwise, but a series of events over long periods of time leads to serious illness. Be patient!

Above all, keep a strong positive attitude and an open mind.

Be perceptive to new ideas.

A NEW LIFESTYLE
WILL EVOLVE.

OUR CHILDREN'S FOOD

A food war has been waged on American soil for more than forty years, the longest chemical war in history. In the past quarter century alone, farmers have dumped over five billion pounds of insecticides onto their crops, more than 11 billion pounds of herbicides onto the soil, and almost 2 billion pounds of fungicides, in an escalating war to ensure good harvests.

Thirty years ago, Rachel Carson in her book, *Silent Spring*, was the first to raise questions about the long-term effects of agricultural poisons on humans. "We have to remember that children born today are exposed to these chemicals from birth, perhaps even before birth. Now what is going to happen to them in adult life, as a result of that exposure? The first generation of children exposed to pesticide residues are now adults. These are the children of the second generation. Only now pesticide use on good crops has increased more than 150 percent. Many child specialists are growing concerned that legal pesticide residues—what are called "tolerances"—have been set for adults. On some foods, those legal residues may be too high for children.

If you're going to be exposed to sort of the same pattern of pesticide residues in the food you eat, you're going to experience a cancer risk by the time you're ten. Dr. Richard Jackson, Environmental Health Committee of the American Academy of Pediatrics said, "If you sit down and you add up what any citizen, but particularly a child, would likely eat and you add up what the government permits in that food, you find out that the government is permitting one hundred, five hundred times as much chemical in the food as a health-based number would dictate."

The Environmental Protection Agency (EPA) is responsible for making sure that 20,000 agricultural products registered for use on food crops are safe. Only two EPA pesticide labs out of thirteen survived the Reagan revolution. Neither is capable of even verifying the pesticide studies that industry submits. All of the tests to prove these chemicals are not hazardous to humans are done by the companies that make them. Can the American people trust the data that comes from an industry that has millions of dollars at stake in the product it's trying to sell? Congress ordered the EPA to make sure the 620 pesticide chemicals then on the market were safe. So far, the EPA has approved the health-safety data for only nineteen. That's just 3 percent. The law ended up creating a bill of rights for older pesticides. It allowed chemicals in use before 1972 to remain on the market until the EPA proves conclusively that they are dangerous. We will continue to be exposed to them, even though the EPA may already have serious doubts about their safety!

Take carrots, for example. Federal law permits the residues of forty pesticides in carrots. The EPA now believes eight may be cancer agents. All of them were registered for use before 1972, and under the law, these old chemicals have special rights. Captan, for example, is a fungicide first registered in 1951. Animal studies have indicated it causes cancer, birth defects, and genetic disorders. Twelve years ago, the EPA began the process of canceling Captan, yet Captan can still be used on seventy-four food crops, including grapes. In fact, the industry's own tests suggest that sixty-five pesticides now in use may cause cancer, but the the EPA can't just ban them until the link is conclusively proven, so their residues remain part of our daily food supply.

But even those tolerances are set for adults. Studies are being conducted on the effect of pesticides, exploring whether the level residues on food are set too high for infants and children. The committee began to amass some shocking data. These levels are not safe for children. Forty percent of our produce comes from outside the country. The third most frequently detected residue is DDT, which is still used heavily in Central America, even though it was banned in this country decades ago. Pesticides are increasingly finding their way into the food chain through fish, birds, and mammals. There are concerns that these pesticide residues are disrupting such basic biological processes as the endocrine, nervous, and immune systems.

We truly don't know what the long-term, cumulative, delayed health effects are of these chemicals in children. If we have 600 active ingredients that are being used in commerce in large, large quantities and we haven't tested but a small subset of them, that means we're using the population as experimental animals for the chemicals we haven't tested. It's outrageous. Every year it goes on without resolution. It's a travesty. We're eating that stuff! Federal law permits the residues of sixty-seven pesticides in strawberries. The EPA suspects that seven may cause cancer. Most of the chemicals sprayed become systemic, meaning they go into the fruit itself.

CHAPTER III

FOOD FOR THOUGHT

We must realize that suggestions for whole foods required by our bodies can cover a wide scope per individual. The foods required for healing can vary greatly with each individual, depending on the illness and stage of crisis.

The food that I am suggesting is only a basic guide.

Green Leafy Vegetables	Beans, Peas, or Grains
Cabbage	Black Beans
Chard	Kidney Beans
Collards	Navy Beans
Kale	Lima Beans
Mustard Greens	Brown Rice
Parsley	Whole Millet
Spinach	Green Peas

Turnip Greens   Chick Peas

Water Cress

Red, Orange or
Dark Purple   Yellow or White

<u>Vegetable</u>   <u>Vegetable</u>

Carrot   Fresh Corn

Red Pepper   Cucumber

Sweet Potato   Radish

Pumpkin   Squash

Tomato   Turnip

Beet   Cauliflower

Eggplant   Avocado

                             Onion

<u>Complete Protein</u>   <u>Green Vegetables</u>

Eggs   Artichoke

Meats   Asparagus

Fish   Celery

Combinations of   Endive

Beans and Grains

Leeks

Okra

Green Pepper

Sprouts

Root Vegetables

Raw Butter

Carrots

Kelp Powder

Potatoes

Sea Salt

Parsnips

Pure Water

Kohlrabi

Turnips

Rutabaga

For eight weeks, choose your breakfast, lunch, supper, and snack menu from the list above. Choose one from each category when planning your plate of seven.

When a food item appears in two categories, only choose it once per meal.

Vegetarians who combine a bean and a grain for their complete protein should choose a separate bean, grain or pea when choosing from the other categories.

Teaspoon-sized portions are recommended for the recovering person with poor digestion.

Tablespoon-sized portions are recommended for the recovering person with adequate digestion.

MAKE SURE TO DRINK PLENTY OF
CLEAN WATER BETWEEN MEALS!

DIGESTION BEGINS IN YOUR MOUTH.

CHEW THOROUGHLY AND ENJOY!

CHAPTER IV

THE BODY'S CRISIS

Common illnesses that are a major link to health-related crises in our bodies at all ages, including childhood, are allergies and asthma. In most cases, excessive mucus buildup any place in our bodies is related to Candida. When we have a Candida development in our bodies, the immune system is compromised and weakened to a great degree.

CANDIDA-RELATED COMPLEX

Contrary to popular thinking, candidacies are not an isolated infectious disease entity but rather a symptom of a disordered immune system. It has characteristics of infection, but there is more to it than that. Invariably other factors are involved, such as food and chemical sensitivities, a reactive hypoglycemic trace-mineral imbalance, accumulations of toxic minerals, an allergy to the yeast itself, emotional and other stresses, and a musculoskeletal imbalance. At a recent candida-update conference sponsored by The International Health Foundation, Inc., it was recommended that, because of its multi-facited ramifications, this condition be referred to as Candida-Related Complex (CRC).

Many readers are already familiar with the precipitating factors in this illness, the most common being repeated use of antibiotics and oral contraceptives, pregnancy, and exposure to toxins. Frequent complicating disorders are parasite infestation, depression of thyroid function, low hydrochloric acid in the stomach, multi-valve prolapse, and chronic viral infections such as Epstein-Barr. Common symptoms are fatigue, food intolerance, digestive disturbances, alcohol intolerance, chronic vaginal discharge, poor memory, depression, chemical sensitivities, premenstrual syndrome, anxiety, emotional disturbance, headache, abnormal weight gain, craving for sweets, and also severe sleeping disorders.

Physical examination of patients with these symptoms ordinarily reveals nothing abnormal. Tests usually produce results "within the normal range." Patients are told, "There is nothing wrong with you."

Because of the complicated nature of this condition, there are no quick and easy answers. Actually, there are answers. But, first all possible causes of the underlying problem must be investigated by means of an integrated evaluation, beginning with a detailed medical history. This should be followed by a comprehensive blood and hair analysis that checks cells for trace minerals and toxic minerals.

An evaluation and digestion tests for food, chemical sensitivities, and other allergies tests of immune system functioning; and other tests such as glucose tolerance test, as needed. Procedures specific for candida are cultures, smears, and blood tests for candida antibodies. Based on all this information, the doctor can, in an alternative medical means, design a treatment plan that leads to relief of symptoms and to optimal health.

Treatment involves an appropriate diet and specific nutritional supplements, according to individual chemical findings. A lactobacillus supplement is necessary for several months to replace the normal bacteria in the intestinal tract.

Diet is the most important aspect of treatment. All "chemicalized" foods and refined sugar products must be avoided. All alcohol, caffeine, tobacco, and foods that obviously contain yeast are to be strictly avoided.

Most patients with CRC are women, but men and children are also affected. In some instances the yeast is passed back and forth between husband and wife. Chronic prosiatitis from yeast can occur and is difficult to eradicate. Many children develop a milk sensitivity, which can result in recurrent middle-ear infections, which are treated with antibiotics, which leads to yeast overgrowth and eventually to Candida-Related Complex. Psychological problems carried as biochemical stresses within the body often prevent patients from getting well until treated with body therapy and psychological counseling.

There is growing evidence that Candida-Related Complex is a common, ubiquitous fact of life. It is essential that physicians realize this and become competent in its diagnosis and treatment, if they are to help the many patients so afflicted.

Evening primrose oil has been shown to be effective in controlling rheumatoid arthritis in a substantial number of people. While the beneficial effects usually take from four to twelve weeks, preliminary evidence suggests that the course of the disease may actually be arrested in some patients. In some studies, for example, in about two-thirds of patients with mild to moderate rheumatoid arthritis, the administration of evening primrose oil seemed to stop the disease process completely.

Eczema is the medical name for skin diseases characterized by inflammation, redness, itching and the exudation of pus. Eczema-like skin disorders are the most frequently reported conditions.

Preliminary studies in several medical research centers used both adults and children, have demonstrated that primrose oil alone has a substantial effect in treating eczema. Results were particularly dramatic for some of the infants. The oil produced complete healing.

"EVENING PRIMROSE OIL HAS BEEN SHOWN TO BE EFFECTIVE IN CONTROLLING RHEUMATOID ARTHRITIS IN A SUBSTANTIAL NUMBER OF PEOPLE."

While experimenting with primrose oil on thousands of people, some unusual and unexpected benefits were repeatedly observed.

The following study illustrates weight loss by people taking primrose oil who made no effort at conscious dieting. Thirty-eight apparently normal individuals took primrose oil capsules over a period of six to eight weeks. Most of the people took four 0.6 mL capsules per day, while a few took eight capsules each day. No effort was made to regulate or change their diets, but some subjects said that they felt less hungry.

Among twenty-two persons who weighed within 10 percent of their ideal body weight, none lost or gained more than five pounds. Of sixteen who weighed more than 10 percent above their ideal body weight, five showed no change, but eleven lost weight. The average weight loss of these eleven people was approximately nine pounds. Four individuals who took eight capsules per day lost eighteen, twenty-two, twenty-four, and eighteen pounds, suggesting that the amount of weight loss was related to the amount of oil

taken. It seems like the answer to a dieter's prayer!

A STAR STILL RISING

The oil of evening primrose will not be the kind of "superstar" that is here today and gone tomorrow. In fact, the star is still rising! The list of research projects on the seed oil of this once lowly flower looks like an international medical who's who! From top research laboratories in South Africa, Canada, the United Kingdom, Argentina, and yes, the United States, dramatic reports are rolling in on the therapeutic effects of evening primrose oil.

The promise of primrose is not confined to therapy as an aid to help those who are sick with any of a variety of conditions. Dr. Horrobin's discovery of evening primrose oil appears destined to rank among the greatest nutritional supplements of preventive medicine of this century.

CHAPTER V

PATHWAYS OF HEALTH

The clear-faced youth grins wholesomely from the small screen. "When I want energy," he says, "I eat a Snickers bar!" Two decades ago, such a claim wouldn't have been taken seriously. Today it is the creed of *millions.*

What is energy, and how do we get it?

Energy has fascinated humanity for centuries. Walt Whitman created some of his most powerful imagery when he wrote; "I sing the body electric; the exquisite realization of health, with the charge of the soul."

"The charge of the soul" describes ancient Chinese teachings on energy. The Chinese viewed energy as "chi," the life-force of the body. Over thousands of years, the Chinese studied the ways man could capture and then harness this energy.

When we think of energy, we think of our "outer" activities: climbing stairs or running to catch a bus. This energy is only the end result of the workings of a miraculous power plant.

Traveling from cell to cell at the speed of light are pulsating currents of pure energy. These cellular power plants supply energy to organs and muscles to keep the body running efficiently.

But we rarely think of this continuous activity within the body. Bodily processes that we take for granted like breathing, cleansing, elimination, fat control, and healing all depend on these countless cellular energy plants.

Our bodies distribute our available energy using strict priorities. Energy goes first to crucial body functions, then to muscles and organs, then digestion, then to cleansing and elimination or healing. But there is only so much energy to go around. Because most people exist at barely half their energy potential, the body must pick and choose. Half of these bodily functions are always being denied.

Fortunately, since our body is a lot wiser than we are, it isn't going to cut off energy for breathing so it can expend the abnormal amount of digestive energy we'll need to digest the typical American meal. Instead, the body will wearily steal that extra digestive energy from elsewhere: "less important" body processes like cleansing elimination, fat maintenance, or organ and muscle tone.

The activity that requires the most energy, and which frequently gets none, is the natural healing processes of the body. Our lifestyles and diets burn up so much energy that our bodies never have any energy left to heal themselves. When our energy supply runs low, all the functions of the body are impaired. Digestion, absorption, assimilation, and elimination drag; circulation and respiration are inefficient. All the tissues and fluids of the body are sluggish. The cells are no longer nourished, and we feel unwell. Health declines. We're sick! This process is called degeneration.

The Four Basic Food Groups

Most of us know that to recharge our energy plants we must eat foods that will provide energy to the body. So we turn faithfully to the four basic food groups: the produce group, the animal group, the processed group, and the sweet or fatty stimulant group.

Today's foods are not produced with nutrition in mind. The concern is often producing foods less expensively and as quickly as possible—at the expense of nutrition.

Our produce is often grown in depleted soil, sprayed with toxic chemicals, placed in cold storage for months…and after just a few hours under supermarket lighting, these so-called fresh fruits and vegetables are depleted of much of their living nutrition. We then go home and cook or boil the rest of it out.

Animal Products

Food products are high in cholesterol and fat and low in fiber, which is the opposite of common sense. This combination extracts a tremendous amount of energy to digest. Lean beef stays in the stomach for up to four hours. Meanwhile, anything else we've eaten with the meat ferments while the body works on digesting the meat. In addition, the animals were raised on diets of "bulking agents," hormones, mold inhibitors, and antibiotics. The result of this foodless diet is passed on to us, which gives the body added stressors to deal with.

The processed food groups are milk products, cereals, chips, noodles, breads, etc. Companies process the vital life energy out of these foods to make them cheaper and more convenient. And forget canned foods. That stuff's dead. These foods may fill us up, but they do little to energize our bodies.

The fourth food group outsells the others by a large margin. The sweet or fatty stimulant group is where most of us turn when faced with an "energy crisis."

This food group offers the glittering promise of instant energy through coffee, soft drinks, cakes, candy, etc. As soon as the temporary surge of "energy" begins to fade, we simply give ourselves another dose. We fall into bed at night dead tired but still wired. By the time our frazzled nervous systems calm down enough to allow sleep, it's time to start over again. The most innocent victims of this food group are the greatest consumers of sweet and fatty stimulants: our children. Destructive life patterns and the foundation for a very unhealthy life are set early.

It has been well established by countless studies that the Standard American Diet is in big trouble. Depending upon our diets for energy is like mining for the gold of pure glowing energy and instead settling for the false glimmer of fool's gold. Empty, depleted foods and stimulants do not adequately feed cells with nutrients to fuel our energy plants. At best, they may only briefly stimulate our nervous systems. (That's why it's called nervous energy.) This gives us a temporary false sense of energy: "fool's energy."

With chronic energy-crisis deficits like this, it's no surprise that an ever-increasing segment of our society is overweight. Is it any wonder we have sluggish fat regulation and organs that aren't doing their jobs?

The body gives us increasingly urgent signals until it finally orders a shutdown of some sort, just to conserve enough energy from our meager store to keep us alive!

The Energy Bank

We have reduced the Standard American Diet to mere chemical or caloric values (as relative as they are), ignoring the basic energy needs of the body.

It's this basic: Everything we put into our mouths either makes an energy deposit or an energy withdrawal. We're healthy when saving and spending are balanced, and we're sick when they're not.

The body doesn't look at food as "calories." It measures food in terms of energetic potential. This occurs in the digestion stage. Everything passes through digestion to be utilized by the body. And digestion takes a great deal of energy. If something we ingest uses up more energy than it gives the body, we are operating at a deficit, and this creates degeneration. Our expanding knowledge of nutrition sometimes inadvertently addresses energy needs. For example, we know that fish is better to eat than beef. Fish also happens to use considerably less energy to digest than beef, therefore giving the body a greater energy deposit.

"THE FREEWAY SYSTEM OF THE BODY"

Traffic Jam

Your car glides onto the freeway, and you settle in for a quiet drive home. But looming ahead, you see cars slowing, and within the next minute, you find that each lane is backed up with cars inching slowly along. Horns blast and tempers flare as an endless stream of cars crawls along bumper-to-bumper. With a sinking feeling, you realize you're going to be delayed for several hours.

For a moment, let's compare the freeway system to the thousands of miles of blood vessels in our bodies. After all, they were both designed for the same purpose: to provide fast, efficient transportation from one point to another. But like the freeways in life, sometimes conditions within aren't as efficient as they could be.

We may have pretty good diets. Even if we eat all the right foods, if these nutrients fail to reach our individual cells, if their crucial mission is impeded at any point along the way, they lose their ability to help us. Think about the nutrients in the foods you eat. These nutrients enter the body with the best of intentions, destined for specific functions of the body. If the digestive system is functioning properly, these nutrients will reach the bloodstream, and if the walls of the arteries are able to absorb the nutrients, they will in turn be carried throughout the body.

But there's trouble in the bloodstream! Each passageway is clogged with plaque, toxins, and deposits slowly inching along. The body sends warning signals to the brain, but the nutrients are going to be delayed. The nutrients we eat find it difficult to reach their destination, if they ever do.

Lifestream of the Body

Blood circulates in the body through a vast, branching network of blood vessels. The bloodstream controls the health of the entire body. A pure, healthy bloodstream enables us to continuously perform these life-sustaining tasks:

- Quick, efficient transportation of life-giving nutrients to waiting cells.

- Effective removal of toxins and wastes from all organs and glands.

- Prompt disease-fighting response.

It's obvious that a sluggish blood circulation system will produce a sluggish and inefficient body. But transportation is just one part of a larger whole. No one system of the body can be separated from the whole. Each system depends upon the others in the complex task of keeping us healthy. For example:

- The lungs supply the blood with oxygen and remove poisonous carbon dioxide.

- The kidneys keep the blood free of poisons, regulating its water and salt content.

- The digestive system breaks food down into chemicals; the blood can then distribute throughout the body.

Within the body's system is a precise cycle of life. After receiving its nutrients, the bloodstream in turn supplies nutrients to each of these systems and organs, as well as each individual cell in the body. These nutrients can then keep the organs functioning so they can supply nutrients to the bloodstream. This cycle depends upon the raw materials we take into our body that feed these processes.

An increasing amount of evidence points at a sluggish system as the cause of many disease conditions. The devil most often named is cholesterol.

Cholesterol Facts

Statistics state that more than 550,000 Americans die each year of coronary heart disease. The evidence is so overwhelming; there can be no doubt of cholesterol's link to heart disease.

But cholesterol is vital to life. It is found in every living cell of the body and is a building block that produces hormones, vitamin D, and digestive bile acids, among other things.

Yet, cholesterol is the principal component of plaque, the fatty, yellowish deposit inside arteries. Plaque accumulates like rust on iron water pipes. Eventually plaque can narrow the arteries enough to severely reduce the flow of blood.

CHAPTER VI

NATURAL HEALING

In our culture, we are apt to be confused by all the pharmaceutical drugs available to us that advertise they capture good health. This healing can never happen when we take prescription mediation, circumventing the body's natural ability to heal itself.

Again, I must remind you that pharmaceutical drugs confuse the body's natural ability to heal itself. The same situation exists to a lesser degree with various health food products, such as vitamins, herbs and the many multi-level marketing products that make many miracle healing claims. So what is the answer to buying the proper health food products?

If we try to become our own practitioners to meet the healing requirements of our body, nothing would happen to heal us. We must have proper guidance in order to buy the products required to help heal our body.

As I have previously mentioned in this book, we must have the basic survival needs such as the cleanest water possible, whole and organic foods (if available), and the cleanest air to breathe.

CHAPTER VII

EXERCISE CAN BE SIMPLE

The requirements for exercise are very simple. It requires only brisk walking and proper breathing for thirty minutes or more daily.

One of the most important things in basic exercise is proper breathing. We breathe not by expanding our rib cage, but by exerting pressure on the diaphragm to force the lungs to work for us. We must learn, during a period of at least fifteen minutes of brisk walking, to exhale and inhale air in equal proportions. One of the biggest problems in our society today is shallow breathing. Proper breathing happens when everything is proportional. Whatever quantity of air we inhale, we must exhale approximately the same quantity. One of the major contributing factors to serious health problems is shallow breathing. This also holds true in weight loss difficulties.

CHAPTER VIII

LOSING WEIGHT

It's no secret: Losing weight is no fun. What's more, after the big battle, gaining it all back can be very frustrating. Why, a person can get discouraged!

Unhappy overweight people become discouraged to the tune of several billion dollars a year—diets, diets and still more diets. Losing weight is a national obsession, and for good reason. Obesity is a threat to our national health.

Obesity will continue to remain a cause for concern until we begin to address its real cause: poor health. That's right. If you're even a little overweight, it's not because you ate too many donuts. It's because your body isn't working at its full capacity.

We've all heard that the only real way to lose weight is to cut calories. Millions continue to hold on to this theory, forcing the body to burn stored calories by taking in fewer calories than are really needed for proper nourishment.

Cutting calories doesn't work. The fact is, we don't gain weight by overeating. Nor do we lose it by under-eating. Consider the millions of people who eat to excess daily and don't gain weight.

Opposing Theories

Nature has this rule: The more we oppose the natural processes of the body, the more the body fights back. Take the immune system, for example.

Our bodies produce antibodies to deal with invading germs. Sometimes when we have weakened energy, we don't produce these antibodies, and we get sick. We then introduce antibiotics into the body, chemicals that do for the immune system what it is not doing for itself. This is fine in the short term; it can save lives.

But there is a problem with this philosophy of substituting for the natural processes of the body. Chemical antibiotics may be killing all sorts of bad germs, but life, when opposed, fights back. When opposed by alien chemical antibiotics, the germs mobilize for a fight. In short, they protect themselves. Use an antibiotic long enough, and it won't even phase the invading germs. You'll have to introduce a new stronger antibiotic. And so it goes.

Fortunately an alternative is quickly gaining popularity. It's called Regeneration. It nourishes the body with the regenerative foods put on the earth to feed a specific system. The body becomes balanced. The body is working. We aren't fighting with ourselves.

The Diet Dilemma

Compare Regeneration to weight loss. Studies have proven that, the more *weight* we try to lose, the more the body will protect its store of fat. We can lose all the weight we want, but the body will hold on to the fat for insurance.

So, we merrily lose "weight," happy that we've lost those final ten pounds but wondering why we look so gaunt in the mirror, why the skin seems to sag, and why we just don't feel very good. Why is this?

Our diet has done this: The weight we've lost is water and protein. **But we still have the fat.** That's all the body has left! It thinks we've been starving it to death. It says defiantly, "Take all the water and protein (skin and body tone) you want, I'm keeping this fat!" Another unhappy dieter is created. There are an awful lot of skinny fat people running around, and they just don't feel good. Why even bother being skinny if you look and feel sick? Nothing (not even lots of curves) is worth poor health. Think about it.

If you're serious about finally losing the fat and doing it right, then it figures since you've made it this far in this book, Doing it right may require some patience, but doesn't anything worth having in life require some patience?

WHAT REALLY HAPPENS WHEN YOU'RE OVERWEIGHT

STARTLING FACTS ABOUT BEING OVERWEIGHT

Sure, being overweight makes you feel uncomfortable and embarrassed about your looks but, the problem of being overweight goes even deeper. So just in case you needed a little extra convincing to start losing weight **RIGHT NOW**, here are some alarming facts.

For every 2 pounds of fat, your body needs one and a quarter extra miles of small arteries just to keep the surrounding tissues alive.

As you gain weight, the skin must stretch to cover the excess bulk. Hence, dry skin, eczema, bruises, and stretch marks are prone to occur.

Excess body weight causes the body to age more rapidly and more visibly.

If you are 20 percent over your normal body weight (that's 24 pounds for a 120 pound woman), your likelihood of living until middle age or beyond is cut by 50 percent.

High blood pressure, a major risk factor for heart attacks and strokes, affects approximately 25 million Americans. Obesity is a chief cause of high blood pressure.

Obese patients are more prone to angina pectoris, a "strangling of the chest." It is a temporary inadequacy in the blood supply to the heart muscle, resulting in shortening of breath and restrictive movement.

Obesity is one of the leading causes of heart attacks, which are the number-one leading cause of death in the United States. The bottom line: obesity is a killer.

Strokes result from bleeding or blood clots in the brain. Obesity is a leading cause of strokes.

As fat builds up in your body, the weight of it causes strain and pain in joints and muscles, resulting in gout and conditions of arthritis.

As you can see, losing weight is crucial to your health, as well as how you look and feel. Make up your mind to start losing weight today. You can lose and maintain your weight with whole foods. You owe it to yourself to look and feel your best!

CHAPTER IX

RULES OF LIFE AND HOW TO USE THEM

WITHOUT CHANGE NOTHING IS POSSIBLE. WITH CHANGE ANYTHING IS POSSIBLE!!!

We don't need drugs!

Healthy Foods and Supplements: No Side Effects

Drugs: Always Side Effects

Have confidence in yourself!

The body has a natural ability to renew itself!

Believe in God—any religion (to be spiritual).

Keep your body and mind in balance with nature.

Now anything is possible!

Those of us who were children in the '30s, '40s, '50s, '60s, '70s or even the early '80s, probably shouldn't have survived.

Our baby cribs were covered with brightly colored lead-based paint. We had no childproof lids or locks on medicine bottles, doors, or cabinets. When we rode our bikes, we had no helmets, not to mention the risks we took hitchhiking.

As children, we would ride in cars with no seat belts or air bags. Riding in the back of a pickup truck on a warm day was always a special treat. We drank water from the garden hose and not from a bottle. Horror!

We ate cupcakes, bread and butter, and drank soda pop with sugar in it, but we were never overweight because we were always outside playing. We shared one soft drink with four friends, from one bottle, and no one actually died from this.

We would spend hours building our go-carts out of scraps and then ride down a hill, only to find out we forgot the brakes. After running into the bushes a few times, we learned to solve the problem. We would leave home in the morning and play all day, as long as we were back when the streetlights came on. No one was able to reach us all day. No cell phones. Unthinkable!

We did not have Playstations, Nintendo 64, X-Boxes, no video games at all, no ninety nine channels on cable, video tape movies, surround sound, cell phones, personal computers, or Internet chat rooms. We had friends! We went outside and found them. We played dodge ball, and sometimes, the ball would really hurt.

We fell out of trees, got cut and broke bones and teeth, and there were no lawsuits from these accidents. They were accidents. No one was to blame but us.

We had fights, punched each other, got black and blue, and learned to get over it. We made up games with sticks and tennis balls, and although we were told it would happen, we did not put-out any eyes. We rode bikes or walked to a friend's home and knocked on the door, rang the bell, or just walked in and talked to them.

Little league had tryouts, and not everyone made the team. Those who didn't had to learn to deal with disappointment. Some students weren't as smart as others, so they failed a grade and were held back to repeat the same grade. Horrors!

Tests were not adjusted for any reason. Our actions were our own. Consequences were expected. The idea of parents bailing us out if we got in trouble in school or broke a law was unheard of. They actually sided with the school or the law. Imagine that!

This generation has produced some of the best risk-takers, problem-solvers, and inventors, ever. We had freedom, failure, success, and responsibility—and we learned how to deal with it.

THE LORD GUIDES US
WITH HIS LOVE, THROUGH
THE POWER OF THE UNIVERSE.

ABOUT THE AUTHOR

I was born on a great day in February 1935.

As life evolved for me, I knew that I had very special aspirations and never-ending dreams of a fantastic life. These dreams were almost shattered at a very young age by a death-defying illness that took several years to recover from. Then the Good Lord gave me my life back with a beautiful future of hope, good health, and happiness. After returning from Korea as a combat soldier, I then entered an aeronautical university and continued my studies in aeronautical science and flight training. Several years later, I landed my first airline job in the former Belgian Congo, flying for the United Nations peacekeeping mission.

After three years in the Congo, I returned to the U.S.A. One and a half years later, I landed a job with Eastern Airlines as a pilot. I am proud to say I had a wonderful twenty-one years with Eastern of which eleven years were as flying captain on many sophisticated jet aircrafts. I then took early retirement from Eastern at forty-eight years of age to sail the vast oceans of our world in my yacht.

It was a warm and beautiful tropical day in Asia during February 1987. That moment stopped my heart. Her name Maria Carmen. Through my lovely wife, I met her aunt, an M.D. from Chicago with more than thirty years of practice in alternative medicine and anti-aging medicine. Working with her, I learned common secrets of self-help and the oriental healing of Regeneration. With my own accomplishments, and regaining my health from serious illness, I feel a true need to share this vast knowledge.

Also, my spiritual belief is of the utmost importance for natural healing. Where there is life, there is hope through change.

Progress is impossible without change, and those who cannot change their minds cannot change anything.

This book is not for self-diagnosis. In the event of illness, contact a health care professional.